# 37 Post Chemotherapy Meal Recipes:

## Get Back On Track with These Nutrient Rich and Vitamin Packed Foods

By

Joe Correa CSN

# COPYRIGHT

This publication is designed to provide accurate and authoritative information in regard to the subject matter covered. It is sold with the understanding that neither the author nor the publisher is engaged in rendering medical advice. If medical advice or assistance is needed, consult with a doctor. This book is considered a guide and should not be used in any way detrimental to your health. Consult with a physician before starting this nutritional plan to make sure it's right for you.

## ACKNOWLEDGEMENTS

This book is dedicated to my friends and family that have had mild or serious illnesses so that you may find a solution and make the necessary changes in your life.

# 37 Post Chemotherapy Meal Recipes:

## Get Back On Track with These Nutrient Rich and Vitamin Packed Foods

### By

### Joe Correa CSN

# CONTENTS

## ABOUT THE AUTHOR

After years of Research, I honestly believe in the positive effects that proper nutrition can have over the body and mind. My knowledge and experience has helped me live healthier throughout the years and which I have shared with family and friends. The more you know about eating and drinking healthier, the sooner you will want to change your life and eating habits.

Nutrition is a key part in the process of being healthy and living longer so get started today. The first step is the most important and the most significant.

# INTRODUCTION

37 Post Chemotherapy Meal Recipes: Get Back On Track with These Nutrient Rich and Vitamin Packed Foods

By Joe Correa CSN

After you defeat cancer, you feel stronger, more powerful, and have a greater urge for a better and healthier life.

After you've finished with chemotherapy, there is one important issue that still remains in your life: how to improve your overall health in the best possible way and enjoy the life ahead of you.

No matter what your the age and gender, the key to a healthier life lies in few basic things: a balanced, diet, exercise, and maintaining a healthy body weight. But, the first and most important thing is a balanced diet. That's the base for a strong recovery after you have dealt with your condition.

In order to help you maintain a balanced diet rich in vitamins, proteins, fibers, etc., I have created a collection of recipes that will give you a quick and easy solution for meals during the post-chemotherapy period.

Every individual has different symptomps after the treatment, but all of them have one thing in common, a delicate organism that needs some fast recovery.

The recipes in this book were created by following a simple rule: the more nutrients, the better. That is what your body needs at this moment, and that is what I want to give you.

You will find an amazing nutritive goldmine in every single one of these recipes. Besides that, they are tasty and good looking which makes them ideal for the entire family!

This wasn't an easy period of life for you. I trully hope these recipes will make the next period of your life better, healthier, and tastier! It is my deepest desire to help you gain back your health and maintain it!

# 37 POST CHEMOTHERAPY MEAL RECIPES: GET BACK ON TRACK WITH THESE NUTRIENT RICH AND VITAMIN PACKED FOODS

### 1. Quick Tuna Salad

**Ingredients:**

2 cups of oil-free tuna, drained

1 small onion, chopped

2 medium-sized red tomatoes, chopped

½ cup fresh parsley, finely chopped

2 tbsp of lemon juice

1 cup of Romaine lettuce, chopped

4 oz of Mozzarella cheese, crumbled

2 tbsp of sour cream, low fat

1 tsp of olive oil

½ tsp of salt

¼ tsp of black pepper, ground

**Preparation:**

Combine the tomatoes, onion, and lettuce in a mixing bowl.

Drizzle with lemon juice and salt to taste. Add tuna and gently toss to evenly distribute the ingredients.

Transfer salad to the serving bowls. Top with sour cream and sprinkle with pepper.

Serve immediately.

**Nutrition information per serving:** Kcal: 380, Protein: 31.4g, Carbs: 18.7g, Fats: 22.4g

## 2. Mountain Sandwiches

**Ingredients:**

1 head of Iceberg lettuce

1 medium-sized tomato, sliced

6 slices of buckwheat bread

**For cream:**

1 tbsp of almonds

2 tbsp of skim milk

½ cup of goat's cheese, crumbled

2 tbsp of walnuts

¼ tbsp of balsamic vinegar

½ tsp of black pepper, ground

½ tsp of salt

1 tsp of chia seeds

**Preparation:**

Combine almonds, walnuts, pepper, and salt in a food processor. Add milk, vinegar, and cheese. Blend until you get a smooth creamy mixture. Transfer to a mixing bowl and stir in one teaspoon of chia seeds. Set aside.

Line one leaf of lettuce and 1-2 slices of tomato onto bread slice. Spread the cream mixture equally over the slice, and cover with another lettuce leaf and bread slice.

**Nutrition information per serving:** Kcal: 143, Protein: 10.4g, Carbs: 21.4g, Fats: 12.4g

## 3. Peppers in Cream

**Ingredients:**

1 cup of Feta cheese, crumbled

1 medium-sized bell pepper, cut into bite-sized pieces

1 tbsp of extra virgin olive oil

2 free-range eggs

½ tsp of salt

½ tsp of ginger

Preparation:

First, boil the eggs. Gently place two eggs in a pot of boiling water. Cook for 10 minutes. Rinse and drain. Cool for a while and peel. You can add one teaspoon of baking soda in a boiling water. This will make the peeling process much easier. Cut the eggs into bite-sized pieces and transfer to a food processor.

Add salt, ginger, and cheese. Blend for 30 seconds or until smooth. Transfer the mixture to a serving bowl.

Add chopped pepper and stir well. Refrigerate for about 30 minutes before serving.

**Nutrition information per serving:** Kcal: 143, Protein: 10.4g, Carbs: 21.4g, Fats: 12.4g

## 4. Winter Frost

**Ingredients**

1 cup of Greek yogurt

1 tsp of coconut flour

1 small peach, halved and pit removed

1 tsp of mint, ground

1 tbsp of honey

1 tsp of red apple zest

½ tsp of vanilla extract

**Preparation:**

Combine all ingredients in a food processor except apple zest, in a food processor. Blend until smooth and transfer to the serving glasses.

Sprinkle the top with coconut flour and apple zest.

Refrigerate at least one hour before serving.

**Nutrition information per serving:** Kcal: 172, Protein: 12.3g, Carbs: 29.5g, Fats: 18.4g

## 5. Wild Blueberry Parfait

**Ingredients:**

½ cup of fresh wild blueberries

2 tbsp of blueberry extract

1 cup of milk

2 tbsp of milk cream

1 large egg

2 egg whites

1 tbsp of honey

**Preparation:**

Gently warm the milk in a large pot over a medium-low temperature. Spoon in the cream and continue to stir constantly. You don't want it to boil! Remove from the heat and set aside to cool for a while.

Add the egg, egg whites, honey, and fresh blueberries. Give it a final stir and refrigerate overnight or at least 3-4 hours before serving.

**Nutrition information per serving:** Kcal: 272, Protein: 12.4g, Carbs: 62.4g, Fats: 18.4g

## 6. Cooked Sea Brass with Horseradish Sauce

**Ingredients:**

2 lb of Sea Brass, boneless

1 medium-sized onion, chopped

2 oz of cherry tomatoes, halved

½ cup of celery, chopped

2 tbsp of fresh parsley, finely chopped

1 medium-sized carrot, sliced

2 tbsp of olive oil

2 garlic cloves, chopped

2 tbsp of lemon juice

1 tsp of vegetable seasoning mix

1 tsp of black pepper, ground

1 tsp of salt

Water

**For sauce:**

1 oz of prepared horseradish

¼ cup of sour cream

1 ts of salt

1 tbsp of capers

**Preparation:**

Place the fish and vegetables into the large pot and pour over water until it covers all ingredients. Add lemon juice, pepper, olive oil, and cover with a lid. Cook for about 30 minutes on low heat. Remove from the heat and set aside to cool.

Meanwhile, combine all sauce ingredients in a mixing bowl. Stir well to combine.

Drain the fish and vegetables and transfer to the serving plate. Drizzle some sauce over the fish and vegetables.

You can serve some lemon slices for extra flavor.

Enjoy!

**Nutrition information per serving:** Kcal: 332, Protein: 32.1g, Carbs: 10.3g, Fats: 13.4g

## 7. Quinoa Prunes Bars

**Ingredients:**

4 tbsp of quinoa, pre-cooked

2 medium-sized bananas, sliced

1 cup of oatmeal

1 free-range egg

1 tsp of cinnamon

1 tsp of flaxseed

½ cup of prunes, finely chopped

1 tbsp of almonds, finely chopped

¼ tbsp of salt

1 tbsp of vegetable oil

Preparation:

Preheat the oven to 400°F.

Combine banana and egg into mixing bowl. Using a fork, whisk well to combine. Set aside.

Take a large mixing bowl and combine all ingredients. Add cooked quinoa and mashed banana-egg mixture. Give it a final stir and transfer to a baking sheet.

Bake for about 25 minutes, or until nicely golden brown. Remove from the oven and set aside to cool for a while.

Cut into equal pieces and serve with milk, but it is, however, optional.

**Nutrition information per serving:** Kcal: 152, Protein: 9.9g, Carbs: 23.5g, Fats: 4.8g

## 8. Potato Bean Salad

**Ingredients:**

3 cups of green beans, pre-cooked

2 medium-sized potatoes, peeled, cubed and pre-cooked

2 tbsp of capers

2 large eggs, pre-cooked, peeled and sliced into wedges

1 tbsp of fresh parsley, finely chopped

**For dressing:**

½ cup of sour cream, low-fat

1 tsp of Dijon mustard

1 tbsp of lemon juice

½ tsp of balsamic vinegar

½ tsp of black pepper, ground

**Preparation:**

Combine all dressing ingredients in a mixing bowl. Stir well to combine and set aside.

Combine beans, capers and potato cubes into a large serving bowl. Top with egg wedges and drizzle with dressing to taste.

For some extra taste, sprinkle with fresh parsley, and serve.

Enjoy!

**Nutrition information per serving:** Kcal: 252, Protein: 8.7g, Carbs: 32.5g, Fats: 10.8g

## 9. Siberian Eggs

**Ingredients:**

6 free-range eggs

½ cup of Circassian cheese, crumbled

½ cup of heavy cream

1 tbsp of fresh parsley, finely chopped

1 tbsp of honey

**Preparation:**

Place two eggs in a pot of boiling water and cook for about 10 minutes. Rinse and drain. Cool for a while and set aside.

Meanwhile, combine cheese, parsley, and heavy cream in a large mixing bowl. Now, peel and cut the eggs into bite-sized pieces and transfer to the creamy mixture.

Top with honey  and refrigerate for 20 minutes before serving.

**Nutrition information per serving:** Kcal: 208, Protein: 13.5g, Carbs: 10.7g, Fats: 13.6g

## 10. Creamed Greens

**Ingredients:**

6 oz of kale, chopped

6 oz of  spinach, chopped

4 oz of Brussel sprouts, halved

2 cups of vegetable broth

½ tsp of black pepper, ground

**For cream:**

2 tbsp od butter

1 tbsp of all-purpose flour

1 tbsp of Dijon mustard

½ cup of sweet cream

1 tsp of salt

½ tsp of red pepper flakes

**Preparation:**

Pour vegetable broth into a deep pot and bring it to a boil. Now, add kale and spinach and sprinkle with pepper for some extra flavor. Add more water if the vegetables are not covered with broth. Cover with a lid and reduce temperature to low. Cook for about 15 minutes, or until soften. Remove from the heat and set aside to cool.

Combine cream ingredients in a mixing bowl. Stir well to combine.

Transfer veggies to a serving plate or bowl, and spoon in the cream. Give it a final stir and sprinkle with some extra red pepper flakes.

Serve immediately.

**Nutrition information per serving:** Kcal: 213, Protein: 5.2g, Carbs: 15.5g, Fats: 14.6g

## 11. Apple Cinnamon Oatmeal Pancake

**Ingredients:**

½ cup of plain flour, gluten-free

1 large egg

1 cup of coconut milk

½ Alfriston apple, grated

¼ cup of almonds, ground

1 tsp of vanilla extract

Cooking oil

Yogurt for topping

**Preparation:**

Combine all ingredients in a large bowl. Spread some cooking oil over a small, non-stick frying pan.

Pour about ½ cup of pancake mixture and cook for about three minutes on each side.

Top with one tablespoon of yogurt.

**Nutrition information per serving:** Kcal:298, Protein:31.4g, Carbs: 42.5g, Fats: 26.7g

## 12. Salmon with Worcestershire Sauce

**Ingredients:**

4 wild salmon steaks, chopped into bite-sized pieces

2 cups of vegetable broth

2 medium-sized carrots, sliced

1 medium-sized zucchini, peeled and sliced

1 medium-sized bell pepper, chopped

**For dressing:**

2 tbsp of Worcestershire sauce

1 tsp of apple cider vinegar

1 tbsp of lemon juice

1 tsp of salt

½ tsp of black pepper, ground

1 tbsp of fresh basil, finely chopped

**Preparation:**

Combine all dressing ingredients in a mixing bowl. Set aside for 15 minutes to allow all flavors to mingle.

Pour 2 cups of vegetable broth into a deep pot. Add salmon chops and vegetables. Season with salt and pepper to taste. Add water if the vegetables are not covered with broth. Cover with a lid and cook for 20 minutes on medium temperature. Remove from the heat and let it cool for a while.

Drain salmon and veggies and transfer to the serving plate. Drizzle with dressing and serve.

Enjoy!

**Nutrition information per serving:** Kcal: 162, Protein: 18.2g, Carbs: 12.8g, Fats: 5.4g

## 13. Blueberry Peach Smoothie

**Ingredients:**

¼  cup of blueberries

1 large peach, pit removed and chopped

1 tbsp of chia seeds

1 cup of almond milk

1 tsp of saliva

**Preparation:**

Combine all ingredients in a blender. Mix until smooth and transfer to a serving glasses. Add some more chia seeds for some extra flavor and nutrients.

Serve!

**Nutrition information per serving:** Kcal: 335, Protein: 28.5g, Carbs: 37.3g, Fats: 10.1g

## 14. Shrimp with Avocado & Eggs

**Ingredients:**

3 cups of shrimps, peeled and deveined

1 medium-sized avocado, ripe

1 ½ cup of brown rice, pre-cooked

2 free range eggs

1 tbsp of honey

2 tsp of olive oil

¼ tsp of red pepper, ground

1 tbsp of red wine vinegar

2 tbsp of sesame seeds

1 cup of red beans, pre-cooked

**Preparation:**

Heat up the olive oil in a large saucepan over a medium temperature. Add honey and stir well until it melts. Now add the shrimps and fry well for few minutes on each side. Season with pepper and remove from the saucepan. Use the same saucepan to fry eggs for about 2 minutes. Transfer to a plate and cut into strips.

In a small bowl, combine the rice with red wine vinegar and red beans. Top with egg strips, shrimps and avocado slices.

**Nutrition information per serving:** Kcal: 246, Protein: 26.5g, Carbs: 6.2g, Fats: 14.7g

## 15. Quick Summer Cold Soup

**Ingredients:**

2 medium-sized tomato, chopped

1 large cucumber, peeled and sliced

1 cup of arugula, chopped

1 tbsp of fresh basil, finely chopped

1 tbsp of fresh coriander, finely chopped

1 cup of buttermilk

1 tbsp of sour cream

½ tsp of black pepper, ground

1 tsp of salt

**Preparation:**

Combine buttermilk, sour cream, salt, pepper, basil, and coriander in large mixing bowl. Stir all well to combine and set aside.

Now, combine tomato, cucumber, and arugula in a food processor. Blend until you get a creamy mixture. Transfer the mixture to the buttermilk bowl and stir all well once again.

Refrigerate for 30 minutes before using.

**Nutrition information per serving:** Kcal: 155, Protein: 8.4g, Carbs: 16.7g, Fats: 8.2g

## 16. Avocado Oil Baked Potato

**Ingredients:**

8 large potatoes, peeled and thickly sliced

3 free-range eggs, hard-boiled

1 cup of cottage cheese, crumbled

2 tbsp of avocado oil

1 tbsp of mustard

1 tsp of salt

½ tsp of red pepper, ground

**Preparation:**

Peel potatoes and cut into thick slices. Cook in boiling water for about 20-30 minutes, until tender. Remove from heat and allow it to cool for a while.

Meanwhile, boil the eggs for 10 minutes. You want hard-boiled eggs for this salad. Peel and cut eggs into slices.

Mix hard-boiled eggs and potatoes in a bowl. Add cottage cheese, avocado oil, mustard, salt and pepper. Stir well with a fork. Cover and chill for about an hour.

You can add ½ tbsp of dried parsley, but this is optional.

**Nutrition information per serving:** Kcal: 351, Protein: 4.7g, Carbs: 37.2g, Fats: 25.8g

## 17. Celery with Dill Sauce

**Ingredients:**

7 oz of celery, cut into lengthwise strips

1 small cucumber, cut into lengthwise strips

1 small zucchini, cut into lengthwise strips

1 medium-sized bulb of fennel, cut into lengthwise strips

1 tbsp of lemon juice

½ tsp of salt

¼ tsp of black pepper, ground

**For the sauce:**

1 cup of Greek yogurt

3 tbsp of vegetable oil

2 tbsp of lemon juice

½ tsp of salt

¼ tsp of black pepper, ground

1 tsp of dill, finely chopped

**Preparation:**

Combine all sauce ingredients in a mixing bowl. Stir well and set aside.

Now, combine all vegetables on the serving plate. Serve sauce from the side, or simply spoon over the veggies.

Season with salt and pepper to taste.

**Nutritional information per serving:** Kcal: 105, Protein: 10.5g, Carbs: 14.6g, Fats: 6.3g

### 18. Wild Green Soup

**Ingredients:**

4 oz of wild asparagus, chopped

2 oz of spinach, chopped

1 tbsp of fresh basil, chopped

2 garlic cloves, crushed

2 tbsp of vegetable oil

1 cup of milk

2 tbsp of fresh parsley, finely chopped

½ tsp of black pepper, ground

½ tsp of salt

Water

**Preparation:**

Combine spinach, milk, basil, and garlic in a blender. Blend until soften and set aside.

Now, place asparagus in a large pot and add one cup of water. Add the blended mixture, and oil. stir all well. Add more water if needed to make a creamy texture. Sprinkle with some salt and pepper. Cover with a lid, reduce the heat to low, and cook for 20 minutes. Remove from the heat and set aside to cool.

Stir in one tablespoon of sour cream for extra sour flavor. This is, however, optional.

**Nutritional information per serving:** Kcal: 105, Protein: 7.7g, Carbs: 13.8g, Fats: 4.5g

### 19. Mediterranean Chicken

**Ingredients:**

2 lbs of chicken breasts, skinless and boneless, chopped into bite-sized pieces

4 garlic cloves, chopped

1 medium-sized onion, peeled and sliced

2 large tomatoes,  chopped

2 tbsp of extra virgin olive oil

1 tbsp of fresh basil, finely chopped

½ tsp of black pepper, ground

½  tsp of salt

1 tsp of vegetable seasoning mix

2 cups of white rice

**Preparation:**

Preheat the oil in a large skillet over medium-high temperature. Add the onion and stir-fry until soften or translucent. Now, add the chicken chops and garlic.

Cook for about 10 minutes or until nicely golden brown color, stirring occasionally.

Meanwhile, place the tomatoes in a food processor.Add a pinch of salt and blend until smooth. Spoon in the mixture into the pan and reduce the temperature to low. Season with pepper. Cover with a lid and cook for 25 minutes. if the mixture too thick, add water occasionally. Remove from the heat and transfer to the serving plate.

Meanwhile, place the rice into the boiling water in a deep pot. Sprinkle with vegetable seasoning mix and cook for 15 minutes. Remove from the heat and drain.

Serve rice with meat and season with fresh basil.

**Nutritional information per serving:** Kcal: 553, Protein: 22.4g, Carbs: 41.2g, Fats: 22.1g

## 20. Oatmeal Soup

**Ingredients:**

4 oz of oatmeal

1 large carrot, sliced

1 cup of celery, sliced

½ cup of parsley, finely chopped

1 small onion, sliced

3 tbsp of vegetable oil

1 tbsp of all-purpose flour

½ tsp of salt

½ tsp of black pepper, ground

½ cup of sour cream

Lukewarm water

**Preparation:**

Preheat the oil in a deep pot over a medium-high temperature. Add the onion and stir-fry until soften. Now add celery, carrot, and parsley and stir well to combine.

Stir in the flour and pour 2 cups of lukewarm water. Sprinkle with some salt and pepper and cover with a lid. Reduce temperature to low and cook for 15 minutes.

Add the oatmeal and check out the level of water. Add more if needed to desired density. Give it a good stir and cook for about 20 minutes more. Remove from the heat and add sour cream. Stir well and leave it for a while to cool.

Serve warm.

**Nutritional information per serving:** Kcal: 85, Protein: 3.2g, Carbs: 14.7g, Fats: 1.7g

## 21. Spanish Omelet

### Ingredients:

4 medium-sized potatoes, peeled and sliced

5 large eggs

1 small onion, diced

2 tbsp of olive oil

1 tbsp of fresh parsley, finely chopped

½ tsp of salt

½ tsp of black pepper, ground

### Preparation:

Beat the eggs in a mixing bowl. Add a pinch of salt, pepper, and parsley and whisk all together. Set aside.

Preheat the oil in large frying pan over a medium-high temperature. Add the sliced potatoes and fry for about 5 minutes, until fork-tender or crisp. Add the onions and cook for 2 minutes more.

Stir in the eggs into the pan and spread equally over the potatoes. Cook for about 3-4 minutes more from both sides. Remove from the heat and slice the omelet into desired shapes or portions.

Serve with tomato slices or some other fresh vegetable.

**Nutritional information per serving:** Kcal: 157, Protein: 9.8g, Carbs: 28.7g, Fats: 3.6g

## 22. Cooked Beets Salad

**Ingredients:**

4 medium-sized beets, peeled and chopped

1 cup of leek, chopped

2 tbsp of lemon juice

1 tsp of salt

½ tsp of black pepper, ground

2 tbsp of olive oil

1 cup of cottage cheese, crumbled

1 small carrot, shredded

1 tsp of parsley, finely chopped

**Preparation:**

Pour 3 cups of water in a large deep pot and bring it to a boil. Gently place the beets and cover with a lid. Reduce the temperature to low and cook until soften, or fork-tender. Remove from the heat and drain. Transfer the beets to the serving bowl.

Now, combine lemon juice, salt, pepper, and oil in a small mixing bowl. Stir well to combine. Set aside.

Add leeks and shredded carrot to the beets and stir well. Spoon in the dressing mixture and give it a final stir. Set aside for about 30 minutes to allow flavors to meld.

Just before serving, add cheese and fresh parsley.

**Nutritional information per serving:** Kcal: 161, Protein: 6.2g, Carbs: 13.4g, Fats: 6.8g

## 23. No-Bake Protein Balls with Oats

**Ingredients:**

1 ½ cup of rolled oats

½ cup of peanut butter

¼ cup of almonds, minced

3 tbsp of honey

1 tbsp of chia seeds,

1 tbsp of vanilla extract, organic

3 cups of milk

**Preparation:**

Place one cup of rolled oats in a bowl. Add other dry ingredients and stir to combine.

Now add in peanut butter and honey. Mix well and gently pour in the milk and vanilla extract.

Shape the balls using your hands, top with the remaining oats and place in the refrigerator for about 30 minutes.

**Nutritional information per serving:** Kcal: 261, Protein: 21.2g, Carbs: 34.5g, Fats: 6.3g

## 24. Brussel Sprouts with Kefir Dressing

**Ingredients:**

1 lb of Brussel sprouts, halved

5 garlic cloves, finely chopped

2 tbsp of olive oil

½ tsp of salt

¼ tsp of black pepper, ground

1 tbsp of butter

**For dressing:**

½ cup of kefir

1 tbsp of lemon juice

½ cup of arugula, finely chopped

½ tsp of salt

1 tbsp of olive oil

**Preparation:**

Preheat the oven to 400°F.

Place the Brussel sprouts in a pot of boiling water. Reduce the heat to low and cook for about 10 minutes, or until soften. Remove from the heat, drain, and set aside.

Melt butter in frying pan over a medium-high temperature. Add garlic and stir-fry until translucent. Add Brussel sprouts and sprinkle with some salt and pepper. Cook for 3 minutes and remove from the heat. Set aside to cool and transfer to the serving bowl.

Meanwhile, combine dressing ingredients in a medium-sized mixing bowl. Stir well to allow flavors to meld.

Drizzle the dressing over the Brussel sprouts and serve!

**Nutritional information per serving:** Kcal: 167, Protein: 6.3g, Carbs: 10.5g, Fats: 14.8g

## 25. Shrimps Spaghetti with Veggies

**Ingredients:**

8 oz of shrimps, peeled and deveined

½ cup of celery, chopped

2 medium-sized carrots, sliced

2 garlic cloves, finely chopped

½ cup of leeks, finely chopped

1 tbsp of olive oil

1 lb of spaghetti (or fresh tagliatelle pasta)

1 tsp of parsley, finely chopped

1 tsp of salt

½ tsp of black pepper, ground

3 tbsp of Parmesan cheese, shredded

**Preparation:**

Use the package instructions to cook spaghetti. When finished, drain, and set aside.

Preheat the oil in a large frying skillet over a medium-high temperature. Add garlic, celery, and leeks. Cook for about

3 minutes and add shrimps. Reduce the heat and sprinkle with salt and pepper to taste. Cook for 5 minutes more stirring constantly. Add 2 cups of and cover with a lid. Cook for 15 minutes or until water evaporates. Remove from the heat and transfer to the spaghetti bowl. Stir in parsley and sprinkle with extra salt and pepper if needed.

Top with shredded parmesan cheese and serve.

**Nutritional information per serving:** Kcal: 220, Protein: 8.3g, Carbs: 44.4g, Fats: 9.8g

## 26. Turmeric Pineapple Smoothie

**Ingredients:**

1 cup of pineapple, chopped

¼ cup of mango, chopped

¼ cup of Goji berries

½ cup of Greek yogurt

1 tsp of turmeric, ground

1 tsp of cinnamon, ground

1 tsp of coconut flour

½ tbsp of honey

**Preparation:**

Combine all ingredients in a blender. Blend for about 1 minute until you get a nice, creamy smoothie. Transfer the mixture to a large serving glasses and refrigerate for about 1 hour before serving.

Just before the serving, you can sprinkle the smoothie with some orange or lemon zest for some extra flavor.

Enjoy!

**Nutritional information per serving:** Kcal: 220, Protein: 5.6g, Carbs: 32.4g, Fats: 1.2g

## 27. Crock Pot Turkey

**Ingredients:**

2 lbs of turkey breast, boneless and skinless, chopped

4 oz of spinach, chopped

1 tbsp of chili powder

2 cups of vegetable broth

2 tbsp of lemon juice

1 tsp of salt

1 tsp of black pepper, ground

2 tbsp of olive oil

**Preparation:**

Preheat the oil in a large pot over a medium-high temperature.

Meanwhile, wash and clean the meat. Sprinkle salt and pepper evenly to coat the meat.

Place the meat chops into the crock pot and cook meat for about 10 minutes. Now, add spinach, chili, and vegetable broth. If needed, pour water to cover all ingredients. Reduce the heat to low and cover with a lid.

Cook for 2 hours. Remove from the heat and leave it to cool.

Just before serving, drizzle the portion with lemon juice.

Place in a crock pot with other ingredients and cover. Cook for about 2 hours.

**Nutrition information per serving:** Kcal: 270, Protein: 35.5g, Carbs: 32.8g, Fats: 24.2g

## 28. Raw Cocoa and Chia Seed Balls

**Ingredients:**

1 cup of minced almonds

½ cup of peanut butter

½ cup of honey

2 tablespoons of minced chia seeds

¼ cup of raw cocoa powder

¼ cup of grated dark chocolate, 85% cocoa

¼ cup of skim milk

**Preparation:**

Combine the ingredients in a bowl and mix well to combine. Shape the balls using your hands and refrigerate for about 30 minutes.

**Nutritional information per serving:** Kcal: 269, Protein: 24.4g, Carbs: 38.2g, Fats:8.5g

### 29. Warm Squid Salad

**Ingredients:**

2 lbs of squids, cleaned, cut into bite-sized pieces

2 tbsp of lemon juice

1 cup of spring onions, chopped

2 medium-sized bell peppers, chopped

3 tbsp of olive oil

1 tsp of salt

½ tsp of black pepper, ground

**Preparation:**

Place squids into a large pot. Add enough water to cover. Cook on a medium temperature for about 15 minutes. Remove from the heat and drain. Transfer the squids to a large bowl.

Add spring onions, peppers, olive oil, salt, and pepper and give it a good stir. Set aside and cover for 2 hours to allow flavors to mingle.

Serve.

**Nutrition information per serving:** Kcal: 302, Protein: 35.2g, Carbs: 46.5g, Fats: 20.3g

### 30. Baked Eggs and Prosciutto in Portobello Mushrooms

**Ingredients:**

6 mushroom Portobello caps, cleaned, de-stemmed, scraped gills

6 strips of Prosciutto

6 large eggs

1 tsp of fresh parsley

3 tbsp of olive oil

½ tsp of salt

1 tsp of black pepper, ground

**Preparation:**

Your mushroom caps should be cleaned and cut into small bowl-like shapes. Take the caps and apply some olive oil on the outside to cook them easily and so that they will not stick to the baking sheet.

Line a baking tray with some baking paper before putting the mushroom caps on them. Take a slice of prosciutto and stuff it inside the mushroom cap. Make sure the slices fits neatly inside it.

Once you have stuffed all your mushroom caps with prosciutto, set them aside. Crack an egg into a small bowl and carefully, slide the egg inside the prosciutto stuffed mushroom cap. This step may take some time since the egg yolk can make the mushroom overturn or spill out.

Once all the eggs are in the mushroom caps, season with some salt, parsley, and pepper. Be careful of the salt since prosciutto is a rather salty meat and adding extra salt might make increase the saltiness of the dish.

Once you have seasoned everything, slide the baking tray extremely carefully into the oven. Be gentle to avoid overturning any mushroom caps. Once they're inside, let them cook for 30 minutes or until you feel the mushroom cap and egg are cooked to your liking.

Let them cool a bit before you take them out of the oven.

Serve:

Serve hot or cold with some sour cream and dill as garnishes.

**Nutrition information per serving:** Kcal: 134, Protein: 14.2g, Carbs: 0.7g, Fats: 7.8g

## 31. Citrus Salmon

**Ingredients:**

1 lb of wild salmon filet, skinless and chopped into bite-sized pieces

3 tbsp of lemon juice

1 tbsp of olive oil

2 tbsp of all-purpose flour

2 oz of butter

4 oz of asparagus, whole

1 tbsp of lime juice

1 tsp of lime zest

1 tsp of salt

1 tsp of black pepper, ground

**Preparation:**

Place meat chops into a large bowl. Add flour, salt, and pepper and coat well using your hands.

Combine butter and oil in a large frying skillet over a medium-high temperature. Heat until butter melts and add meat chops. Cook for 15 minutes, or until golden brown. Transfer the meat to another dish and reserve the pan.

Add lemon juice, lime juice, and asparagus to skillet and cook for 5 minutes, stirring occasionally.

Return the salmon chops to the pan, add salt and pepper, and stir all to combine. Cook for 5 minutes and remove from the heat. Transfer all to a serving plate.

Top with a pinch of lime zest and serve.

**Nutrition information per serving:** Kcal: 282, Protein: 42.1g, Carbs: 7.5g, Fats: 12.2g

## 32. Wild Berries Pancakes with Rice Flour

**Ingredients:**

1 cup of mixed wild berries, fresh

½ cup of rice flour

½ cup of skim milk

½ cup of almond milk

3 tbsp of honey

1 tsp of organic vanilla extract, powdered

1 tsp of baking powder

1 whole egg

½ cup of low-fat cream

½ cup of agave syrup

1 tbsp of sunflower oil

**Preparation:**

Combine flour, baking powder, skim milk and almond milk in a bowl and mix well with a fork, until smooth mixture.

In another bowl, mix the cream with 3 tbsp of honey, vanilla extract, and egg. Beat well with a fork, or even better with an electric mixer. You want to get a foamy mixture.

Whisk in this mixture in a first bowl to make a thick batter.

Cover it and let it stand for about 15 minutes.

Heat a tablespoon of sunflower oil in a non-stick frying pan.

Use ¼ cup of pancake mixture to make one pancake. You can use some pancake molds, but this is optional.

Fry your pancakes for about 2-3 minutes on each side. This mixture should give you 6 pancakes.

Spread 1 tbsp of agave syrup over each pancake, top with wild berries and serve.

**Nutrition information per serving:** Kcal: 312, Protein: 38.1, Carbs: 42.4g, Fats: 25.5g

### 33. Tagliatelle in Melon Sauce

**Ingredients:**

1 lb of Tagliatelle pasta, pre-cooked

1 small melon, peeled, seeds removed and chopped

2 oz of butter

1 cup of sweet cream

½ tsp of salt

½ tsp of black pepper, ground

1 tsp of vegetable seasoning mix

¼ cup of Parmesan, shredded

1 tbsp of fresh parsley, finely chopped

**Preparation:**

Use the package instructions to cook pasta. Drain well and transfer to a large bowl.

Meanwhile, combine melon chops and sweet cream in a blender. Blend until smooth creamy mixture. Set aside.

Melt butter in a large frying skillet over a medium heat. Add melon cream mixture, salt, pepper, and vegetable seasoning mix. Pour ½ cup of lukewarm water and stir constantly. Cook for 10 minutes and remove from the heat.

Pour the sauce over the pasta and top with shredded Parmesan and parsley.

**Nutrition information per serving:** Kcal: 293, Protein: 9.6g, Carbs: 63.7g, Fats: 15.8g

## 34. Brussels Sprouts in Coconut Gravy

**Ingredients:**

1 lb of Brussels sprouts

2 cup of coconut milk

4 onions, chopped

1 tbsp of olive oil

½ tsp of salt

½ tsp of black pepper, ground

½ cup of cashew paste

1 tbsp of fresh coriander, finely chopped

Preparation:

Heat up some olive oil in a large frying skillet. Add the onions and stir-fry for several minutes. Now add the Brussels sprouts and cashew paste. Reduce the heat to medium and fry for about 5 minutes.

Add the coconut milk, season with some salt and pepper and cover. Cook for about 10 minutes over a medium-low temperature.

Remove from the heat and top with the fresh coriander.

**Nutrition information per serving:** Kcal: 123, Protein: 4.5g, Carbs: 10.6g, Fats: g

## 35. Spicy Vegetable Minestrone

### Ingredients:

4 oz of green beans, halved

2 medium-sized carrots, sliced

1 cup of celery, chopped

1 cup of white beans

1 large zucchini, peeled and sliced

1 medium-sized onion, sliced

3 tbsp of vegetable oil

3 garlic cloves, chopped

1 tsp of fresh basil, chopped

1 tsp of chili, ground

1 tbsp of cayenne pepper, ground

1 tsp of fresh rosemary, crushed

1 cup of tomato sauce

1 tbsp of fresh parsley, finely chopped

1 tsp of vegetable seasoning mix

## Preparation:

Preheat the oil in a deep pot over a medium-high temperature. Add garlic and onion and stir-fry for 2 minutes. Now add carrot, green beans,white beans, zucchinis, and celery. Sprinkle with salt and pepper and pour water enough to cover all ingredients. Cover with a lid and reduce the temperature to low. Cook for about 15 minutes and add tomato sauce and all remaining spices.

Cook for 1 hour and remove from the heat. Open the lid and let it cool for a while.

Just before serving, sprinkle with some fresh rosemary for extra taste.

**Nutrition information per serving:** Kcal: 120, Protein: g, Carbs: 63.7g, Fats: 15.8g

## 36. Apple Cinnamon Oats

**Ingredients:**

½ cup gluten-free oats

1cup of water

1 Alkmene apple, peeled and grated

1 apple, sliced

2 tbsp of almond yogurt

1 tsp of cinnamon, ground

**Preparation:**

Boil the water and add oats. Briefly, cook (for several minutes) and reduce the heat.

Add one grated Alkmene apple and one teaspoon of cinnamon. Simmer for another ten minutes. Remove from the heat.

Top with almond yogurt and sliced apple. Serve warm.

**Nutrition information per serving:** Kcal: 120, Protein: 3.5g, Carbs: 25.8g, Fats: 1.3g

## 37. Rice Pasta with Homemade Salsa

**Ingredients:**

1 pack of rice pasta

3 large ripe tomatoes

1 tbsp of olive oil

2 garlic cloves, crushed

½ tsp of dry oregano

¼ tsp of salt

**Preparation:**

Use the package instructions to prepare pasta. Rinse well and drain. Set aside.

Peel and roughly chop the tomatoes. Make sure you keep all the liquid.

Heat up the oil over a medium temperature. Add the garlic and stir-fry for several minutes.

Now add tomatoes, oregano, salt, stevia, and oregano. Reduce the heat to low and cook until the tomatoes have softened.

Add ¼ cup of water and cook for 10 more minutes stirring constantly.

Turn off the heat, add pasta and cover. Let it stand for 10 minutes before serving.

You can use the olive oil instead of butter, but I prefer the butter because it gives a nice, soft taste. Serve it with grated smoked cheese, grated Parmesan, crushed garlic, finely chopped parsley, or whatever you like.

**Nutritional information per serving:** Kcal: 390, Protein: 12.4g, Carbs: 44.3g, Fats: 26.4

# ADDITIONAL TITLES FROM THIS AUTHOR

70 Effective Meal Recipes to Prevent and Solve Being Overweight: Burn Fat Fast by Using Proper Dieting and Smart Nutrition

By

Joe Correa CSN

48 Acne Solving Meal Recipes: The Fast and Natural Path to Fixing Your Acne Problems in Less Than 10 Days!

By

Joe Correa CSN

41 Alzheimer's Preventing Meal Recipes: Reduce or Eliminate Your Alzheimer's Condition in 30 Days or Less!

By

Joe Correa CSN

70 Effective Breast Cancer Meal Recipes: Prevent and Fight Breast Cancer with Smart Nutrition and Powerful Foods

By

Joe Correa CSN

9 781635 312096